CROHN'S DISEASE

NATURAL HELP and ADVICE

Author: Sheila Ber –
Naturopathic Consultant.

CROHN'S DISEASE HELP and BEST ADVICE – My Personal Successful Regimen.

MY SIMPLE AND BEST ADVICE TO YOU:

<u>Vitamin D3</u> deficiency is a major factor for Crohn's. I personally take 8,000 - 10,000 I.U. a day, divided by two, 2x a day.

Try like myself taking the above dosage, but always with a spoon of Flax or Fish oil, to optimize absorption. Vitamin D will give you energy, reduces inflammation, balances your Thyroid, and other hormones, protects you against developing cancer, maintains healthy nervous system, helps you sleep better, and much more.

Eliminate sugars and replace with Honey in everything! Honey is comprised of mono-saccharides, and easily digested by Crohn's afflicted bowels, therefore less bacterial growth that causes inflammation. Try also to take 1/2 tsp of MANUKA HONEY, on empty stomach 1 hour before a meal.

This honey heals any wound inside and outside the body!!! It contains Hydrogen Peroxide and other beneficial properties that speed healing.
If you are allergic to fructose, do not eat honey! Try Stevia.

MANUKA honey is a product of New Zealand.

*Please note: If honey isn't stored properly, or comes in an inadequate packaging, it is vulnerable to bacterial contamination. It may be stored at room temperature, always with the lid properly closed.

It helps against any abdominal pain! I tried it when I had pain from Crohn's attack, the pain was gone. The cost is about $12.00 for small jar, and it lasts for a reasonably long time.

SUGAR IN ANY FORM, IS EXTREMELY HARMFUL TO THE INFLAMED BOWELS OF CROHN'S SUFFERERS.

Try to avoid smoking, and coffee, only once a day or every other day! Instead of coffee, to be alert and awake, put a dash or two of CAYENNE PEPPER into 1/2 cup of warm water, or into salads, soups, any dishes. It does wonders! It also takes pain away!!!

Taking daily: 2 Tablespoons of APPLE CIDER VINEGAR in 1 cup of warm water, helps tremendously! Absolutely!
Take also fruit PECTIN powder – ½ tsp in 1 cup warm water. It alleviates irritation in the bowels, and heals.

Pectin is very beneficial for healthy colon and helps to fight Arthritis, Diabetes, High Cholesterol, high blood pressure and much more. It is also a blood purifier.

I take also 1 coated baby Aspirin 81 mg. every day, or every other day. It keeps inflammation down, and the blood thin, due to high ESR associated with Crohn's disease.

It prevents potential strokes in older adults, due to associated high blood Platelets count, and high ESR (Erythrocyte sedimentation rate).

You will not regret implementing the above suggestions, as you are getting them from a Crohn's sufferer like yourself, who is mature in years, and with experience, and who has tried everything. I have provided in this book, many helpful suggestions for emergency situations. If you don't try, you'll never know...

Check with your G.P. your thyroid level, and Hemoglobin level as well.

You might need Iron pills (best from vegetable source). www.vitacost.com sells them at a reasonable price - Item #CTL4026594. Take 3 a day with vitamin C - 500-1000 mg, for 3 months.

When in intense pain, for immediate relief, take also 1 tablespoon Colloidal Silver, but swash in the mouth for a few seconds, then swallow. In 5-7 minutes, the pain subsides.

Additionally take: <u>ROBERT'S COMPLEX</u> Enzymatic therapy (in Canada the cost is approx. $20.00). It is extremely helpful to avert an attack.
Take it 3x a day, for several days only, on an empty stomach until you feel better.

Crohn's pain, any abdominal pain, can be alleviated effectively also, with boiled (5 min.) herbal concoction:

Sage, Mint, Anise. Drink warm, several times/day. It's very healing and detoxifying. Don't forget the MANUKA HONEY also for the pain!

<u>Don't</u>: eat fried food!

<u>Don't drink raw milk!</u> You must minimize drinking milk. You can drink 2-3 cups a week, but <u>you must boil it first!!!</u> Because milk has a specific bacteria that severely aggravates Crohn's condition. If you boil it, you should have no problem.

<u>Do not</u> drink alcohol, as all alcoholic drinks contain yeast. Yeast overgrowth is toxic, damaging, and can cause inflammation.

When you consume <u>yeasty foods and drinks</u>, such as: PIZZA, PASTRY, WINE, BEER, consume in moderation, and immediately take Probiotics, to get rid of the yeast in your body, before it gets out of control. Probiotics also digest and kill yeast. Yeasty foods can cause addiction.

Do eat: 2-3x a week SALMON fish, and also chicken. These are healing to the bowels, and anti-inflammatory. They are beneficial for the heart, brain, and for depression as well.

Take: Cod liver oil: 2-3 tablespoons daily. It is anti inflammatory, and keeps your blood vessels in good shape. It also helps ward off depression.

Eat rice daily if you can, until you get better. When you feel better, you can increase your potatoes and bread (whole wheat or 7 grains) intake. Rice is the only complex carbohydrates that best agrees with Crohn's afflicted bowels. You can cook it in many different ways.

You can even add raisins, slivered almonds, add 3 tablespoons of honey, 2 tablespoon Grape seed oil (best oil) and 1/2 teaspoon butter, nutmeg, some cinnamon, grated lemon peel (1/3 teaspoon), 1/2 cup milk, or condensed milk (in a can).
Bring to a boil, and simmer for about 15 minutes. Eat cool or warm.

- *8* -

The worst thing that you can do is to feel sorry for yourself. I know Crohn's can cause depression. But you have to try to remain strong, positive, and hopeful! You must move on with life.

You have to be flexible when it comes to food, and give up the items that cause you trouble (inflammation).

* If you make a mistake and you eat something you shouldn't, or if stress causes you an attack, despite all efforts, don't give up! Keep fighting it, and try all the tips given to you in this book.

It takes time to heal, and slowly you will heal, I promise! However, you have to make some changes, you just have to, or you could suffer big time.

Try and visualize your intestines, and what you put into them!

Always take HONEY to substitute sugar! Also MANUKA HONEY for <u>pain</u>. Take also PROBIOTICS ("Primal Defense" is best!) to keep microbial level, and inflammation down.

If you are allergic to fructose, do not eat honey! Most people are not allergic to honey.

Remember: that the intestines can heal at any moment, slowly and surely. It takes 3-5 days for the intestinal tissue to heal, if you eat the right food.

However, you have to control what you eat, and how much. Again, just try to look inside you. Stay calm, try not to worry.

If you feel depressed, you must take B-Complex 2-3 times a day, and L-Theanine (amino acid) 1-2 capsules a day. You may drink coffee, no more than once a day, as it can aggravate the inflammation in your bowels. However, at the same time, coffee is beneficial in elevating your Serotonin level, making you feeling content).

To fight depression and inflammation, take also two (2) to four (4) tablespoon cod liver oil daily. The oil is extremely helpful, and has many health benefits. It contains Vitamin A&D, also EPA and DHA. It coats the bowel tissue to prevent irritation cause, by anything that you eat or drink.

If you fancy Chinese food, it can be oily! Veggies and rice, that are not oily, are OK. Soya sauce can aggravate Crohn's, so try to stay away from it. You can add 1-2 spoons of Olive oil when frying your food.

Orange is also very aggravating. Instead of lemon use lime, as it feels better for the Crohn's bowels. It is less acidic.

Chicken Teriyaki has soya sauce and it can aggravate. Steak is good, potatoes are OK, with added olive oil topping them, some parsley, lime juice and salt, it's all healing and excellent tasting.

Eggs - *I find that if you eat them 3 times a week, and then rest 2-3 days, alternately, your body is less likely to develop intolerance (allergy) for eggs. But then it is individual.*

White flour in any form or shape (bread, cakes, cookies etc) can be harmful for Crohn's, especially when high inflammation present. You can try some when you start to feel better.

I eat whole wheat bread, or 7 grains, but keep it to minimum, because the flour converts to sugars (polysaccharides and disaccharides,) and the bowels have difficult time digesting them. I take enzymes to help with that.

Complex Carbohydrates such as rice is all right. (Basmati is best!).

Potatoes, are all right, if eaten 2-3 times a week. Due to their high starch content, the bowels can have difficult time digesting them. Always take enzymes just before any meal.

Sandwich with home cooked meat is OK, but definitely <u>not the cold cuts!</u> Cold cuts will cause an immediate attack, and more inflammation as a result. The bowels can react very negatively, including the forming of intestinal blockage. The preservatives in the cold cuts: Sodium Nitrate & Sodium Nitrite, are carcinogenic, and are also very aggravating to the Crohn's afflicted bowels.

<u>Don't eat</u>: Apples, oranges, or pizza, only after your bowels are healed.

<u>Do eat</u>: Bananas (excellent! even 2-3x a day), broccoli is very good, but must be washed and boiled for 3-5 minutes, to make it easier on the bowels to digest. Carrots are very good, but until your bowels get better, you must cook the carrots for about 5 minutes, for easier digestion.

Tomatoes are very good, but can irritate your sensitive bowels. You may eat fresh tomatoes with sprinkled Olive oil on top, and a dash of Oregano.

It tastes great. The Olive oil coats the bowels, preventing the acidity of the tomatoes from interacting with them.

Pizza - 1-2 slices are OK, but because of the yeast in the crust, you must take 2 capsules of PROBIOTICS immediately, in order to prevent any yeast damage to your bowels. Probiotics will digest and kill the yeast.
If you fail to do that, you may experience pain and bloating, also increase in inflammation.

Pancakes are Ok, if you eat 2-3, and only with HONEY. You can add Cinnamon, or nutmeg for flavour.

Do not use any syrup, not even Maple syrup, due to the high sugar content (disaccharides) that can further damage the bowels.

You can obtain tasty, non pasteurized honey in the Health store. A popular brand in Canada is: Dutchman`s Gold. 1 Kg is as low as $9.00 plus tax.

Please bear in mind that:
*Inflammation and pain is the result of, as shown in the following equations:

INCREASED STRESS + ACIDIC DIET + TOXINS = INCREASED BODY ACIDITY = LOW ACIDIC pH.

INCREASED ACIDITY = HIGHER MICROBIAL LEVEL.

HIGHER MICROBIAL LEVEL = MORE TOXINS = INCREASED INFLAMMATION AND PAIN!

RELAXATION + SLIGHTLY ALKALINE DIET + TOXIN ELIMINATION = DECREASED BODY ACIDITY = SLIGHTLY ALKALINE pH.

<u>DECREASED ACIDITY = LOWER MICROBIAL LEVEL = BALANCED INTESTINAL FLORA = DECREASED INFLAMMATION AND PAIN! = OPTIMUM HEALTH!</u>

<u>ALKALIZE DAILY!</u>

HOW TO ALKALIZE YOUR BODY: **The simplest, most economical way to alkalize: 1/2 tsp Baking Soda in 1 cup water, daily. If you are very acidic, the above can be done two times a day.**

GOOD LUCK!

SHEILA BER, 2013.

DISCLAIMER.

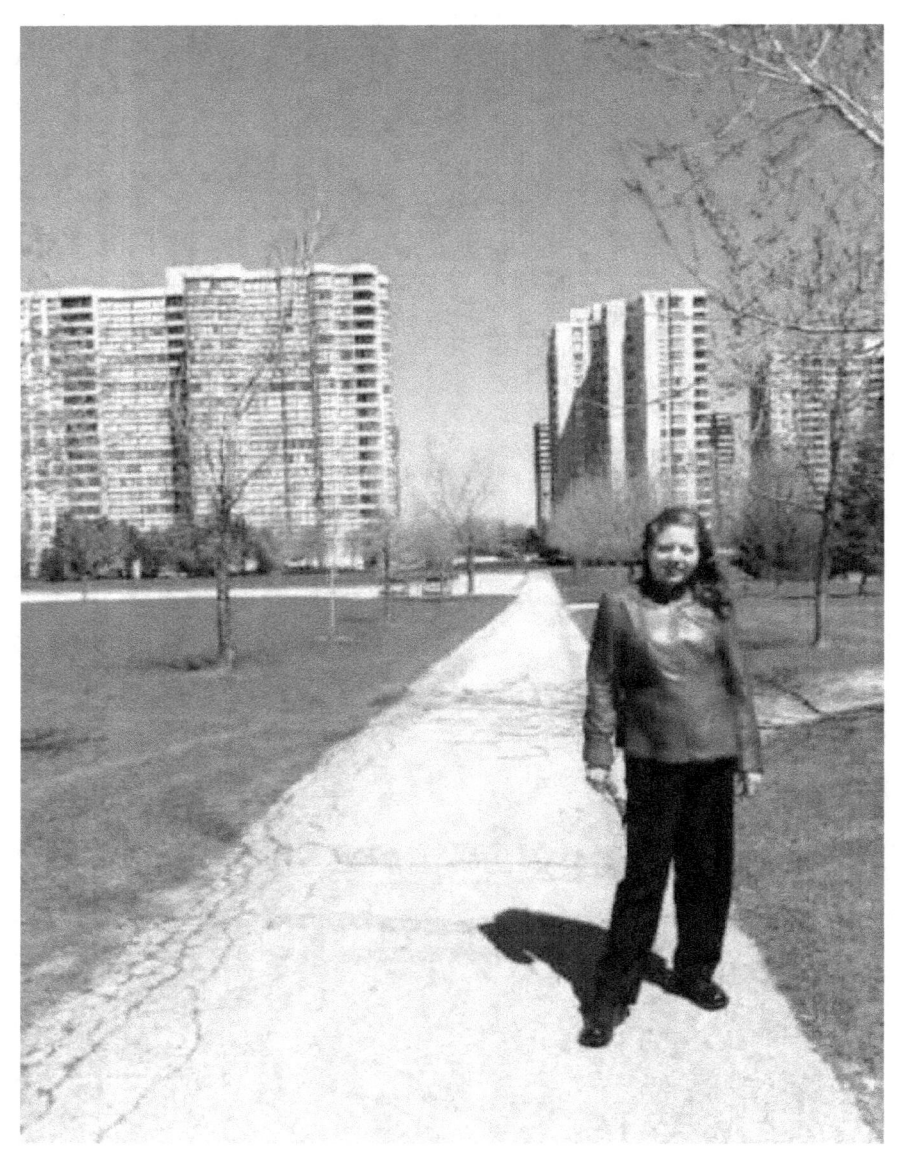

SHEILA BER, 2013.
(SHULLA)

See the following books written also by Sheila Ber:
1. *"Alkalize & Survive"*
2. *"Insomnia – Natural Treatment"*
3. *"Arthritis – Help & Advice*
4. *"The pH Connection"*
5. *"Eat Well and Lose Weight"*
    at:
    www.Amazon.com
    www.Createspace.com
    www.Kobobooks.com
    www.Indigo.Chapters.ca

SHEILA BER BIOGRAPHY   2012.

Professionally:

I'm a **Microbiological/Chemical Technologist**, currently working as a **Naturopathic consultant**.
I worked in Microbiology and Chemistry, for about 12 years, in the Pharmaceutical, cosmetics, and toiletry industries.

I started out as a microbiological/Chemical Analyst. I Performed: chemical and microbiological analysis of raw materials, finished products, variety of packaging materials and their compatibility with different range of finished products.

Chemical analysis tests were carried out with up to date technologically advanced instruments, such as Spectrophotometers, and other apparatus.
Microbiological tests including incubation of samples, and microscopical studies of a variety of bacteria, yeast, and fungus.

I was also involved in Research & Development, and in formulations of large variety of products.
I've carried out many formulations, and modified some when required.

My work included:

1) Quality Control of raw materials, finished products, packaging.

2) I was responsible for managing and supporting the laboratory personnel.

3) Additionally, I have carried out inspections on the production floor facilities, the equipment, including ventilation system, and other systems. Monthly reporting on the findings, my recommendations, and implementation of required corrective actions.

4) Communication with Health Canada, particularly to obtain their regulatory approvals for new patents and new products. Providing them with documentation, and MSDS information of the raw material involved, in all the formulations.
I have tremendously enjoyed all the above duties.

It's very technically involved work, very interesting, and challenging.

Personally:

Generally, I'm rather unconventional, though as getting older, I become slightly more conventional. I like things straight, simple, and uncomplicated.
I like helping people. I try to view things, situations, from different perspectives.

I refrain from judging others, but need to know all the facts and reasons for their particular behaviour, thoughts and actions, before forming any opinion.
I take everything with a grain of salt, always stay alert, and cautious.

Life has its highs and lows, but I always try to stay afloat. Trying is the key word!

I often check my expectations, and keep them in perspective.

I have two grown up sons. I love them very dearly.
I enjoy being a caring mother, not perfect, and with always room for improvement.

EDUCATION:
I've graduated with **Honours in Science,** *and with* **Distinction in Physics.**

Seneca College
Microbiological/Chemical Technology

Technical school
Architecture/Mechanical Drafting

School of Accounting
General Accounting

OCCUPATION:

I'm currently working as a Naturopathic Consultant.

EMPLOYMENT HISTORY:
DRUG TRADING COMPANY - Toronto
Microbiological/Chemical Technologist

FABERGE - Toronto
Quality Control/ Laboratory Manager

REVLON - Toronto
Quality Control/ Laboratory Manager

ACCENTURE Business for Utilities - Toronto
Accounting/Administration

I **Lived in:**

1) Toronto, Canada,
2) Argentina, Buenos Aires.